Janaice Vitória Dias Lima
Antonio da Costa Cardoso Neto
Márcia Silva de Oliveira

SELF-CARE FOR PEOPLE WITH DIABETES MELLITUS

Janaice Vitória Dias Lima
Antonio da Costa Cardoso Neto
Márcia Silva de Oliveira

SELF-CARE FOR PEOPLE WITH DIABETES MELLITUS

TYPE 1

ScienciaScripts

Imprint
Any brand names and product names mentioned in this book are subject to trademark, brand or patent protection and are trademarks or registered trademarks of their respective holders. The use of brand names, product names, common names, trade names, product descriptions etc. even without a particular marking in this work is in no way to be construed to mean that such names may be regarded as unrestricted in respect of trademark and brand protection legislation and could thus be used by anyone.

Cover image: www.ingimage.com

This book is a translation from the original published under ISBN 978-620-6-76194-5.

Publisher:
Sciencia Scripts
is a trademark of
Dodo Books Indian Ocean Ltd. and OmniScriptum S.R.L publishing group

120 High Road, East Finchley, London, N2 9ED, United Kingdom
Str. Armeneasca 28/1, office 1, Chisinau MD-2012, Republic of Moldova, Europe
Printed at: see last page
ISBN: 978-620-8-34453-5

SUMMARY

INTRODUCTION **3**
OBJECTIVES **5**
GENERAL OBJECTIVE 5
SPECIFIC OBJECTIVES 5
LITERATURE REVIEW **6**
METHODOLOGY **27**
RESULTS AND DISCUSSION **30**
CONCLUSION **38**
REFERENCES **40**
AUTHORS' BIOGRAPHIES **45**

INTRODUCTION

According to the World Health Organization (WHO), type 1 diabetes mellitus (DM1) is a chronic condition in which the pancreas does not produce enough insulin. Insulin is crucial for glucose to enter cells and be converted into energy. In this type of diabetes, the immune system attacks and destroys the beta cells of the pancreas, which are responsible for producing insulin (World Health Organization, 2022).

In this sense, it's important to note that type 1 diabetes includes the following symptoms: intense thirst, increased urinary frequency, extremely intense hunger, unexplained weight loss, fatigue and blurred vision. Usually diagnosed in childhood or adolescence, type 1 diabetes can appear at any age. Treatment consists of insulin application, regular monitoring of glucose levels, a balanced diet and regular physical activity (WHO, 2022).

From this context, it is understood that studying type 1 diabetes mellitus is of extreme social, academic and professional importance since it is a chronic disease that affects millions of people worldwide, including many children and adolescents. Deepening knowledge about DM1 can contribute to the development of more effective treatments, improvements in patients' quality of life, and a significant reduction in health system costs. In addition, education and awareness about DM1 are key to challenging stigmas and promoting a supportive environment for those living with the condition, enabling greater social inclusion and more effective support.

This study seeks to answer the following guiding question: What is the impact of self-care on the health of individuals with Type

1 Diabetes Mellitus? In this sense, the study aims to carry out a systematic review on the importance of self-care for individuals with Type 1 Diabetes Mellitus. In order to answer the objectives proposed in this work, the following topics will be discussed: diagnosis, treatment, the importance of nursing in care and health education in the self-care of individuals with type 1 diabetes mellitus. In addition, the methodological path will be presented with the flow diagram, results with discussions and conclusion of the study.

OBJECTIVES

GENERAL OBJECTIVE

- Carry out a systematic review on the importance of self-care for individuals with Type 1 Diabetes Mellitus.

SPECIFIC OBJECTIVES

- Learn about the challenges of diagnosing and treating type 1 diabetes mellitus;
- To describe the importance of nursing in caring for individuals with DM1;
- To identify the influence of health education on the self-care of individuals with Type 1 Diabetes Mellitus.

LITERATURE REVIEW

DIAGNOSIS AND TREATMENT OF TYPE 1 DIABETES MELLITUS

Type 1 diabetes mellitus (DM1), formerly known as juvenile diabetes, accounts for 10.0% of all cases of diabetes. This chronic disease is characterized by absolute insulin deficiency and its causes are related a autoimmune processes triggered by the interaction of genetic and environmental factors. This disease can occur at any age, but is usually diagnosed before the age of 20. Complications can lead to early disability and reduced quality of life, as well as economic losses caused by high medical costs and frequent hospitalizations (Nass, *et al.*, 2019).

This disease usually progresses in a progressive way that can have serious consequences for the health and well-being of individuals and also imposes high costs on health and social systems. According to the WHO, the prevalence of diabetes is increasing and is currently considered the pandemic of the 21st century. It is estimated that the disease will affect more than 20% of the world's population in the next 20 years, with the global prevalence of diabetes doubling since 1980, from 4.7% to 8.5% among adults (Santos, 2023).

Currently, there has been a considerable increase in the rate of type 1 diabetes mellitus, which is the result of various social, economic, demographic, environmental and genetic factors. Around 1.1 million young people live with DM1. Research shows that Brazil is the country with the highest number of new cases diagnosed in children up to the age of 14, and health education is key to controlling the disease (Dutra,

et al., 2023).

Due to changes in dietary patterns and changes in the profile of the world's population in recent decades, the nutritional status of children and adolescents with DM1 is similar to that of healthy people, although a high prevalence of overweight and obesity can also be observed in this group. Lifestyle changes resulting from reduced dietary restrictions through more flexible insulin therapy and lower energy consumption, facilitated by more screen time with electronic devices such as television and video games, contribute to obesity (Silva, Silva, Oliveira, *et al.,* 2020).

The age-related differences, as well as the metabolic, genetic and immunogenetic properties of DM1 require an individualized approach for each individual, because in addition to the variable loss of insulin secretion, residual insulin production (detectable C-peptide) also tends to be higher, which occurs more frequently in adult DM1 than in juvenile DM1, while diabetic ketoacidosis occurs more frequently in young people with this disease (Reis, *et al.*, 2023).

DM1 is a type of diabetes commonly diagnosed in children, adolescents and, in some cases, young adults and affects men and women equally. It is a chronic, multifactorial autoimmune disease caused by the partial or complete destruction of the beta cells of the islets of Langerhans in the pancreas, leading to insufficient insulin production. It can take months or years to reach this point. Usually the onset of the disease is sudden and in 1/3 of cases the first manifestation is diabetic ketoacidosis. As it is a serious metabolic disorder, it must be treated in a hospital environment (Smaniotto; Pascolat, 2022).

Early diagnosis of DM1 is crucial for patients' health and well-being. Identifying the disease in the early stages allows appropriate treatment to be started, avoiding serious complications such as diabetic ketoacidosis, a potentially fatal condition. In addition, early diagnosis helps stabilize blood glucose levels, reducing the risk of long-term damage to the body's organs and systems, such as the kidneys, nerves, eyes and heart. This provides a better quality of life and a longer life expectancy for individuals with DM1 (Ramalho, *et al.,* 2024).

In addition to the clinical benefits, early diagnosis of DM1 also has a significant psychological and emotional impact on the patient and their family. Knowing about the condition early on makes it possible to educate and adapt to a new lifestyle, including dietary changes, constant glucose monitoring and insulin administration. This adaptation process is made easier with adequate support from health professionals, who offer guidance and psychological support. With an accurate and timely diagnosis, it is possible to manage the disease effectively, promoting an active and healthy life for those with DM1 (Hermes *et al.*, 2021).

It is essential to be aware of the changes caused by the disease that can result in complications. However, it is common for these complications to stand out in relation to other changes, such as foot deformities, changes in the way you walk and skin dryness, which can be detected early and treated (Mendonça, *et al.*, 2022).

Experiencing type 1 diabetes in childhood or adolescence is a difficult experience that generates conflicts and difficulties due to the unpredictability of the disease, as well as the demands and changes in lifestyle that require treatment. From the moment of diagnosis, treatment can be complicated because it involves many daily tasks that impact on family dynamics, as well as barriers to therapeutic integration due to clinical and sociodemographic factors that can influence the child's state of health (Ramalho, *et al.*, 2024).

The difficulties associated with type 1 diabetes in adolescence are greater because this disease demands maturity, responsibility and self-care from adolescents given its chronic nature. In addition, adolescents must understand that they have to live with certain limits and boundaries, as the diagnosis of type 1 diabetes requires them to adapt to a new lifestyle (Zanatta, *et al.*, 2020).

It is important to remember that the shock of the diagnosis, changes in habits and self-care have a direct impact on the patient's mental health. As part of the treatment of insulin-dependent DM1, various measures should be recommended such as: daily insulin injections, maintaining normal blood glucose levels, daily dietary care, medical consultation, regular physical exercise and strategies to overcome any problems (Maniotto; Pascolat, 2022).

It is noteworthy that psychological and social factors are included as important for evaluation in the treatment of DM1. It is also important to highlight the need to assess emotional factors, such as depression, anxiety and stress, when there is a decrease in glycemic control, as they are very important for monitoring treatment (Melo, *et al.*, 2019).

DM1 has a significant effect on children's quality of life, especially with regard to social isolation due to the feeling of inferiority in relation to other children. They also have difficulty adapting to new habits such as studying and playing and tend to have emotional problems (Smaniotto; Pascolat, 2022).

It is a disease that is difficult to control and prone to various acute and chronic complications. Therefore, once the diagnosis has been confirmed, it is necessary to carry out rigorous, long-term treatment to ensure adequate nutrition, controlled physical activity and insulin therapy. Limited access to medication, negligence in monitoring blood glucose and unhealthy lifestyles can lead to the patient's death (Pedrinho, *et* al., 2020).

Faced with this diagnosis, adolescents must change their habits and lifestyle, especially those related to blood glucose control and the implementation of a healthy lifestyle, such as a balanced diet, regular physical activity and adherence to drug treatment when necessary (Zanatta, *et al.*, 2020).

The treatment of DM1 raises a number of additional concerns because the disease mainly affects children and adolescents. Attention must be paid to sexual maturity, physiological changes and physical growth; these changes are common and alter insulin conversion and lead the student to learn about self-care from the beginning of the diagnosis (Smaniotto; Pascolat, 2022).

People with this type of diabetes depend on insulin and need to be administered this hormone. Treatment aims to prevent chronic complications at the microvascular level such as nephropathy and retinopathy, as well as macrovascular complications such as stroke, while reducing the risk of acute illnesses such as severe hypoglycemia (Reis, *et al.*, 2023).

A medical condition called DM1 presents symptoms such as mood swings, nausea, vomiting, fatigue, weakness, weight loss even with excessive food intake, constant thirst and frequent urination. To treat this condition, five main components are needed: education, the use of insulin, glucose monitoring, nutritional guidance and encouragement to exercise. Treatment is complex and requires the participation of the family, who must also accompany the patient to consultations with the health team (Jesuíno, 2021).

It aims to control diabetes and prevent chronic complications. It involves changes in daily life that involve adopting habits, including: continuous blood glucose checks; healthy food; reducing the use of industrial products; daily practice of at least one physical activity and administration of medication at a certain time (oral antidiabetic and/or insulin) (Melo, *et al.,* 2019).

As for the importance of adherence to non-drug treatment, a review study found that aerobic exercise had a significant impact on heart rate and blood glucose control when adhering to a diet. Appropriate treatment ensures that blood glucose does not change suddenly, thus reducing the need to seek medication to control it (Santos, *et al.*, 2020).

Adherence to treatment for chronic diseases such as DM1 makes a difference to the lives of children, adolescents and their families. This requires lifestyle changes, which include, in addition to dietary restrictions, the need for physical exercise and painful procedures such as checking capillary blood glucose and frequent insulin administration (Souza, *et al.*, 2020).

Faced with this therapeutic need, family members, especially caregivers, must acquire specific knowledge about the composition of food, signs and symptoms of hypoglycemia and hyperglycemia, and be trained in the preparation and administration of medication (Souza, *et al.*, 2020).

The identification of significant relationships between the results tested and various indicators of organizational access allows us to conclude that the effectiveness of help for people with diabetes is related to actions other than those proposed by the ESF team during the treatment itself. This includes, for example, arriving or scheduling a medical appointment on the same day as the search for the UBS and waiting time at the location (Santos, *et al.,* 2020).

It is important to consider that a late diagnosis or non-adherence to DM1 treatment can lead to the development of other complications and diseases, including visual, renal, pancreatic and cardiovascular alterations (Brito, *et al.*, 2020; Guzman, 2021).

In order to maintain stable blood sugar levels, diabetes treatment requires children to live a more disciplined life. Considering the chronic nature of this disease, which will accompany children throughout their lives, it is important to develop health strategies that contribute to greater knowledge about this disease and its treatment (Pedrinho, *et al.*, 2020).

Living with DM1 requires young people to adjust their lifestyle, self-control, acceptance and resignation. However, awareness of this need can only be achieved as adulthood develops and taking into account the stage of the disease and its context. Thus, the responsibilities previously attributed to carers are gradually being taken over by the younger generations, who are trying to adapt to a new lifestyle. In this context, it is important to promote self-care practices, taking into account the need to understand the patient's condition and assess the factors that influence their treatment (Nass, *et al.*, 2019).

In order to avoid the serious consequences of this chronic disease, it is essential that patients take care of their own well-being, adopting preventive measures such as being able to manage their medication, following dietary guidelines and exercising daily. These attitudes promote a change in habits and encourage the adoption of a healthier lifestyle, contributing to the control of the disease (Rodrigues, *et al.,* 2022).

A IMPORTANCE OF NURSING IN CARE OF INDIVIDUALS WITH TYPE 1 DIABETES MELLITUS.

The nursing process is a methodological tool developed in five interrelated phases (history, diagnosis, planning, implementation and nursing evaluation) that guides professional nursing care. Its development must be supported by a theoretical framework that guides professional practice and registration. When carried out in outpatient clinics, at home, at school, in community associations, among others, the nursing process is equivalent to a nursing consultation, precisely because the nurse develops all the interconnected stages in a single moment (Rosa, *et al.*, 2021).

The nursing diagnosis arises from a complete assessment of the patient and includes limiting stress factors and strengthening lines of defense, after which interventions are planned to strengthen these lines of resistance at different levels: primary, secondary and tertiary. Nursing interventions at any level of prevention are designed to support the system in its adaptation or adjustment, maintaining a certain level of stability (Santos, *et al.*, 2023).

There are currently several strategies for developing self-care activities aimed at DM, ranging from activities that require mediation with technological devices, such as phones and software, to tools for assessing a person's knowledge and attitudes towards the different characteristics of the disease, such as the Diabetes Knowledge and Psychological Attitudes Questionnaire, a tool that can help establish educational strategies for self-care, individualize and improve tools for managing the disease (Hermes *et al.*, 2021).

Nursing plays an important role in caring for patients with DM1, a chronic disease that requires continuous and careful management. Nurses are often the health professionals closest to patients, providing fundamental support in monitoring blood sugar, administering insulin and educating them about self-care. This proximity allows for quick and effective intervention in the event of hyperglycemia or hypoglycemia, thus helping to stabilize the patient (Zanatta, *et al.*, 2020).

The emotional support of nurses is another important aspect of caring for patients with DM1. Living with a chronic illness can be difficult and stressful, and caregivers are trained to provide psychological and motivational support. This support can make a significant difference in the patient's adherence to treatment and in maintaining a healthy lifestyle (Rodrigues, *et al.*, 2022).

Nurses also play an important role in coordinating multidisciplinary care. Patients with DM1 often require care from several health professionals, including endocrinologists, nutritionists and psychologists. The nursing team ensures that all parts of the treatment are integrated and promotes a holistic approach that meets all the patient's needs (Dutra, *et al.*, 2023).

Nursing research has also had a significant impact on improving care for patients with DM1. Nursing researchers explore new management and education strategies, thus contributing to the development of better clinical practice. The results of this research are often integrated into treatment protocols, thus improving the quality of care (Mendonça, *et al.*, 2022).

Advocacy is also an important part of the nurse's role in caring for patients with type 1 diabetes. Nurses often advocate on behalf of patients, ensuring that they have access to the necessary resources and that their rights are respected. This advocacy can range from fighting for better health policies to ensuring equal and fair treatment for patients (Hermes *et al.*, 2021).

In addition to practical tasks, the nurses educate patients and their families about type 1 diabetes and provide detailed information about nutrition, exercise and the importance of regular blood sugar monitoring. Education is essential to enable patients to manage their disease independently and effectively. Through educational sessions, caregivers help demystify diabetes management and reduce the fear and anxiety associated with the diagnosis (Merino, *et al.*, 2022).

Nurses caring for children with DM1 should look for educational strategies that encourage the child to be aware of their condition and to make an effort to look after themselves. The technical procedures for maintaining DM1 can be reproduced without the individual really knowing what they are doing. In this context, although children are aware of the need for treatment, they often seem unable to clearly assess the risks and complications that the inappropriate application of procedures can bring to their health, and it is up to family members to guide them in this regard (Pedrinho, *et al.*, 2020).

The integration of professionals in primary health services and hospitals, as well as collaboration between the two, is also a concern when determining the interventions to implement. Before surgery, school nurses should undergo training involving the pediatric multidisciplinary team and the hospital's primary care multidisciplinary team (Dixe, *et al.*, 2020).

Nursing interventions in community care, with the consequent transfer of knowledge, therapeutic care relationships and teamwork, are centered on communication. This process involves the exchange of information that can influence individuals and communities to improve health and prevent disease (Santos, 2023).

Healthcare providers must be prepared to assess the educational, behavioral, emotional and psychosocial factors that interfere with the development of a treatment plan and work collaboratively with the child and family to address barriers and prepare them for self-care (Hermes *et al.*, 2021).

The health needs of children and adolescents affected by DM1 include special daily attention to the disease itself and the resolution of potential emergencies. And in order to increase the independence and autonomy of children/adolescents, communication between health professionals and school nurses is very important (Santos, *et al.*, 2023).

Early diagnosis and adherence make it possible to control DM and its complications. The nursing consultation is one of the strategies used for monitoring and health education for the purposes of disease control. In this context, nurses face challenges in providing direct and indirect care to individuals, families and communities. It is up to nurses to develop this support and raise awareness of the need for lifestyle changes required in the treatment plan (Rosa, *et al.,* 2021).

It's up to the nurses, who are part of the multidisciplinary team, to administer the first dose of insulin. This will also help to reinforce the guidelines and encourage children to gain independence in using their own insulin, always under the guidance and supervision of an adult. I have observed that the insecurities and fears of adults are overcome by the courage and very rapid adaptation of children with these comorbidities (Jesuíno, 2021).

Nursing plays a key role in health education with the aim of controlling DM1. Nurses are often the first health professionals to interact with newly diagnosed patients and their families and provide initial advice on how to treat the disease. They are responsible for teaching important skills such as insulin self-administration, blood sugar monitoring and dietary adjustments. This initial training is very important for patients to feel empowered and confident in managing their disease (Mendonça, *et al.*, 2022).

In addition to initial training, nurses play an ongoing role in the management of type 1 diabetes. They hold regular meetings to monitor the patient's progress, adjust treatment plans and provide additional advice if necessary. During these meetings, nurses can identify compliance issues, answer questions and help resolve any problems the patient is facing. This continuous monitoring is important for maintaining good glycemic control and preventing complications (Guzman, 2021).

Nurses also play an important role in educating patients about the prevention and treatment of acute complications of type 1 diabetes, such as hypoglycemia and diabetic ketoacidosis. They teach patients to recognize the signs and symptoms of this condition, as well as the appropriate actions to treat it. This knowledge is key to reducing the number of medical emergencies and improving patient safety. In addition, nurses can educate patients about the importance of having regular check-ups to detect chronic complications of diabetes early (Zanatta, *et al.*, 2020).

Health education carried out by nurses is also tailored to patients' individual needs. When developing an educational plan, factors such as age, level of understanding, social and cultural background and personal preferences are also taken into account.

For example, for children and adolescents, nurses can use interactive and fun approaches to make learning more accessible and engaging. This personalization is important to ensure that health education is effective and relevant for each patient (Reis, *et al.,* 2023).

Nurses also play an important role in training family members and caregivers of patients with DM1. They provide guidance on how to support patients in the day-to-day management of the disease, including insulin administration, meal planning and recognizing signs of complications. Educating family members and healthcare professionals is especially important for younger or older patients, who may be more dependent on the support of others to effectively manage the disease (Santos, et al ,.'2023). In addition to directly educating patients and their families, nurses also collaborate with other healthcare professionals to ensure integrated and comprehensive care. They can work closely with endocrinologists, nutritionists and psychologists to develop and implement a treatment plan that addresses all all aspects of treatment of

DM1. This multidisciplinary approach ensures that patients receive comprehensive support and
coordinated (Dixe, *met al.,* 2020).

Nurses also play an important role in promoting a healthy lifestyle in patients with DM1. They provide advice on the importance of regular exercise, a balanced diet and stress management strategies. A healthy lifestyle is an important part of diabetes management and nursing support can help patients adopt and maintain these practices over time (Smaniotto; Pascolat, 2022).

Finally, health education provided by nurses should be considered a continuous and dynamic process. As new research and technologies emerge, nurses must continually update their knowledge and skills to provide the best advice to patients. This includes keeping abreast of new treatments, glucose monitors and other diabetes innovations. In this way, nurses ensure that patients have access to the latest tools and information to manage their disease effectively (Merino, *et al.*, 2022).

Nursing intervention in emergency situations involving patients with DM1 is essential to ensure a rapid and effective response capable of saving human lives. When patients with DM1 show signs of severe hypoglycemia, such as mental confusion, loss of consciousness or convulsions, nurses must act immediately, administering intravenous glucose or glucagon if necessary. The ability to quickly recognize symptoms and initiate appropriate interventions is key to preventing serious and life-threatening complications (Rodrigues, *et al.*, 2022).

In addition to hypoglycemia, nurses also play an important role in treating attacks of diabetic ketoacidosis, which is a serious complication of DM1. Diabetic ketoacidosis is characterized by severe hyperglycemia, ketonemia and metabolic acidosis. The nurse should carefully monitor the patient's vital signs, as well as glucose and ketone levels, and start administering intravenous fluids and insulin (Santos, 2023).

According to studies, nursing professionals also play an important role in monitoring possible complications, such as electrolyte and glycemic imbalances, and in communicating with other members of the healthcare team to ensure complete and coordinated treatment (Dixe, *et al.*, 2020).

In addition to clinical interventions, nurses have an educational role to play in emergency situations. They should explain to patients and their families the root causes of these crises, such as insulin administration errors or infections, and advise them on how to prevent future emergencies. This learning includes the importance of regularly checking blood sugar levels, recognizing the first signs of decompensation and knowing when to seek medical attention. By providing this educational support, nurses help patients to better manage their type 1 diabetes and reduce the risk of future emergencies (Jesuíno, 2021).

It should be emphasized that understanding the treatment will make it possible for health professionals to develop appropriate coping strategies, making the child more participative and enabling the acquisition of self-care skills (Pedrinho, *et al.*, 2020).

HEALTH EDUCATION IN THE SELF-CARE OF INDIVIDUALS WITH TYPE 1 DIABETES MELLITUS

In order for individuals to achieve positive results and a good prognosis, clear communication between doctor and patient is necessary, as well as an understanding of the instructions received during the medical consultation. Individual self-management of diabetes is essential for better health outcomes and there are important factors that can influence adherence to treatment, including commitment and clarity of communication, understanding of treatment needs and the importance of adherence (Rodrigues, Matos, Tenani, *et al.*, 2022).

Health education efforts based on the needs of the subject and carried out in a dialogical, participatory and systematic way can have a positive impact. In this way, it leads to a better level of knowledge among children and adolescents about how to manage the disease properly and improves their ability to take care of themselves, for example when using insulin (Hermes *et al.,* 2021).

Health education plays an important role in the fight against DM1, a chronic disease that requires ongoing treatment. It provides patients and their families with the knowledge and skills to treat the disease effectively. Through educational programs, patients learn the importance of regular blood sugar monitoring, proper insulin administration, a balanced diet and exercise. This knowledge allows for greater autonomy and security in the face of the disease (Brito, *et al.*, 2020).

In addition to daily management, health education also includes understanding the signs and symptoms of acute complications, such as hypoglycemia and diabetic ketoacidosis. Well-informed patients will be better able to recognize these situations more quickly and act appropriately to prevent or treat them early. This reduces the frequency of medical emergencies and hospitalizations and improves the quality of life of patients with DM1 (Marques, *et l.,* 2019).

Health education is not limited to patients, but also includes training family members and caregivers. It plays an important role in daily support, especially for children and the elderly with DM1. Adequate training of health professionals in aspects such as insulin administration, proper food preparation and recognizing signs of complications can significantly improve disease management and patient safety (Guzman, 2021).

Health education in the context of DM1 should be an ongoing process, keeping pace with changes in patients' lives and advances in medicine and technology. With the emergence of new therapies, monitoring devices and health apps, it is important that patients and their families stay informed. This ensures that they can make the most of these innovations for better diabetes control, reduced complications and improved quality of life in the long term (Rosa, *et al.*, 2021).

To adopt self-care behaviors, the individual must first be convinced that their disease is dangerous to them and can cause serious harm, that the behaviors adopted are effective in managing and controlling the disease, and that there are difficulties in carrying out self-care actions. specific implementations and behaviors are not worth the benefits (Nass, *et al.*, 2019).

However, certain behaviors require technical and cognitive skills and these are generally associated with self-efficacy beliefs. Therefore, as self-efficacy influences the person to perform or not perform bad behaviors and overcome obstacles that may arise, it should be encouraged by health workers through educational activities (Nass, *et al.*, 2019).

The availability of information, from the diagnosis of DM1 to treatment, makes it possible to advocate and engage the public about their health concerns. The complexity of these living conditions calls for better health education. In this case, there are technological tools that facilitate the promotion of health education for people with DM1, the understanding of the disease and its treatment and the strengthening of self-care (Dutra, *et al.*, 2023).

Therefore, diabetes education implies the need for an individual and family learning process that encourages the progressive monitoring of the development of the child's autonomy in taking charge of their own care (Pedrinho, *et al.*, 2020).

Educational materials should be designed to help the healthcare team communicate, supporting the verbal information provided to child patients and their families, and providing guidance on care in an organized manner, which helps to avoid contradictory information. It is essential to ensure that not only printed materials are delivered, but also that communication between health professionals is effective, with sharing of experiences in which everyone is active in the construction of knowledge (Hermes *et al*., 2021).

Health education encourages individual and family responsibility in managing the promotion and treatment of DM1. Communication is the most important individual empowerment tool. To this end, professionals should opt for an individual-centered approach, as scientific literature shows that individual treatment is effective in stimulating change and achieving good metabolic control (Dutra, *et al*., 2023).

Health workers must be able to carry out dialogical and reflective educational activities that improve the cultural level of society, as well as the professionals involved, in order to improve their counseling and communication skills (Mendonça*, et al*., 2022).

In the context of the pediatric population, educators of children with DM1, regardless of the level of care, are encouraged to develop educational technologies that facilitate their work processes and reinforce them with playful resources. These resources allow professionals to use their technical-scientific knowledge to exchange knowledge in order to improve the quality of the services provided (Dutra, *et al*., 2023).

The role of health literacy in controlling blood sugar and blood pressure is very important, because individual health behavior and routine use of health services are very important in controlling risk factors. In addition, the treatment of these chronic diseases depends on the individual's skill set and ability to understand the information provided by the healthcare team and the data needed to monitor the progression of the disease, take medication and change lifestyle and diet (Rodrigues, *et al.,* 2022).

Also according to Rodrigues, *et al.* (2022), a higher level of health education is linked to better control of chronic diseases, such as diabetes, due to the understanding of health information. This results in a more positive prognosis for patients. Therefore, this approach is essential to promote health and prevent short- and long-term complications related to diabetes.

Increased health education leads to changes in habits, as deficiencies in the management of the ingredients needed to control glycemia can cause problems and affect the glycemic profile of those suffering from diabetes. By ensuring safe behavior and taking due care in the proper handling and use of insulin, satisfactory measures can be achieved, as insulin's action as a hypoglycemic hormone in the blood is essential for the quality and maintenance of human vitality (Dutra, *et al*., 2023).

However, processing errors can be a common problem and have a direct impact on blood sugar profiles. By ensuring safe behavior, reasonable therapeutic measures and adequate insulin use, satisfactory glycemic control indicators can be achieved (Merino, *et al.,* 2022).

Health education efforts based on the needs of the subject and carried out in a dialogical, participatory and systematic way can have a positive impact. In this way, it leads to a better level of knowledge among children and adolescents about how to manage the disease properly and improves their ability to take care of themselves, for example when using insulin (Hermes *et al.*, 2021).

Health education plays an important role in the fight against

DM1, a chronic disease that requires continuous treatment.

This provides patients and their families with the knowledge and skills to treat the disease effectively. Through educational programs, patients learn the importance of regular blood sugar monitoring, proper insulin administration, a balanced diet and exercise. This knowledge provides greater autonomy and confidence in managing the condition (Brito, *et al.*, 2020). In addition to daily treatment, health education also includes understanding the signs and symptoms of acute complications, such as hypoglycemia and diabetic ketoacidosis. Well-informed patients will be able to to recognize these situations more more quickly e act appropriately to prevent or treat them at an early stage. This reduces the incidence of medical emergencies and hospital admissions, thus improving the quality of life of patients suffering from DM1
(Zanatta, *et al.*, 2020).

Health education is not just limited to patients, but also includes training family members and health professionals. It plays an important role in day-to-day support, especially for children and the elderly with type 1 diabetes. Adequate training of nursing staff in aspects such as insulin administration, preparing appropriate meals and recognizing signs of complications can significantly improve disease control and patient safety (Guzman, 2021).

Health education in the context of DM1 should be an ongoing process that takes into account changes in patients' lives and advances in medicine and technology. With the emergence of new therapies, monitoring devices and health apps, it is important that patients and their families stay informed. This ensures that they can make the most of these innovations to better manage their diabetes, reduce complications and improve their quality of life in the long term

(Rosa, *et al.,* 2021).

It is recommended to carry out intensive and practical educational programs on diabetes, including theoretical parts on knowledge about the disease, nutrition, physical exercise, insulin and hypoglycemia, self-analysis, self-management, macro- and microvascular complications and practice. This part, which includes technical training (self-monitoring and self-care, insulin injection, carbohydrate counting) and practical training (preventing hypoglycemia and taking action when it occurs, adjusting insulin doses, planning exercise), proved to be very effective at six months and intervention one year later (Nass*, et al., 2019),* 2019).

METHODOLOGY

This is a systematic review of the importance of self-care for individuals with type 1 diabetes mellitus.

The following databases were used in this study: MEDLINE (Medical Literature Analysis and Retrieval System Online), BDENF (Nursing Database) and LILACS (Latin American and Caribbean Health Sciences Literature). To facilitate access to the database searches, the BVS (Virtual Health Library) regional portal was used. The descriptors were chosen according to DeCS (Health Sciences Descriptors) and MeSH (Medical Subject Headings). In accordance with the DeCS and MeSH list, the terms used were: "Type 1 Diabetes Mellitus", "Self-Care" and "Health Care". In addition to the descriptors, the Boolean operators "AND" and "OR" were used to combine the terms in the databases.

During data collection from the databases, a flow chart was constructed to clarify how the articles included in the study were selected. To analyze the data, a composite table was built identifying the authors, year of publication, title of the article, database, type of study and relevant results. The results were interpreted and analyzed based on a synthesis of the results, comparing the data found in the articles included in this study.

We followed the recommendations of the PRISMA statement, which consists of a checklist of 27 elements and a flow diagram to help authors improve the communication of the review (Moher *et al.*, 2009; Urrútia; Bonfill, 2010; Cardoso Neto, Oliveira, 2023). The data for this study was collected from the databases between February and July 2024, with the aim of answering the following guiding question: What is the impact of self-care on the health of individuals with Type 1 Diabetes Mellitus?

According to the databases, 2,311 articles were identified, in which we found: 1,203 articles in MEDLINE, 981 articles in LILACS and

127 articles in BDENF. First, 1,984 were eliminated using the following filters: full text, language - Portuguese, period 2019-2024. A total of 337 articles were selected. Subsequently, 59 duplicate articles were excluded, leaving 278 selected articles; 246 articles were excluded by title and abstract, 32 full articles were selected for final eligibility; of these 20 full articles were excluded from the analysis because they did not contemplate the objective of the study, 12 articles were included in the study as observed in the flow diagram, constructed for the process of selecting scientific articles.

Inclusion criteria were original articles published in Portuguese in the previous five years, which addressed the topic to be studied and allowed full access to the study content. Non-inclusion criteria were articles eliminated by filters, incomplete articles published before 2019, duplicate articles, articles excluded by title and abstract that did not meet the objective of the study, complete articles were excluded from the analysis after careful reading that were not available in full.

What stands out in the current study is the author's interpretation and personal critical analysis that led to the inclusion of the articles for the study. The author has chosen materials with information that appropriately considers the study as presented here and that meets his expectations.

Figure 1: Flow diagram of the article selection process scientific

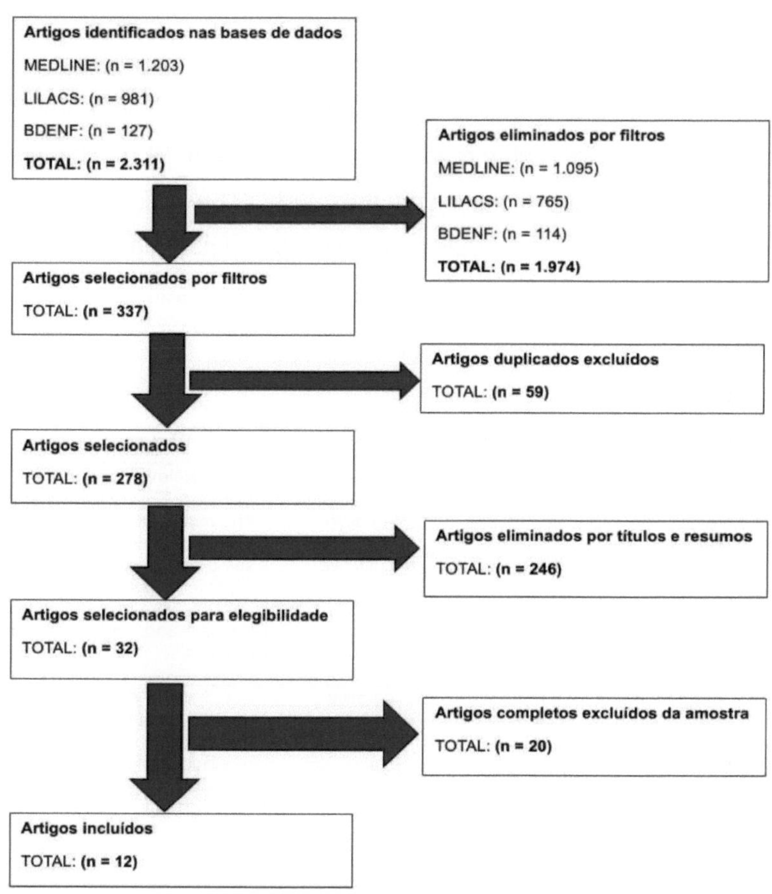

Source: Author.

RESULTS AND DISCUSSION

Table 1 shows an overview of the number of articles that were analyzed and included for this systematic review study. In the study, 32 articles were thoroughly read and analyzed, and 12 articles were selected for definitive inclusion in the study. The articles selected include: Authors, year of publication, title, the database from which they were selected, type of study and the relevant results as shown in Table 1:

Chart 01 - Articles used in the systematic review.

NO.	Author/Year	Title/Databases	Type of study	Relevant results
01	Almeida; Santos; Santos, (2023)	The importance of for patient self-care. LILACS	Integrative review with a quantitative approach	The results of this study demonstrate the importance of health education in self-care, with a significant improvement in quality of life, as patients were trained to manage their illness and health costs were reduced.
02	Araújo, Melo, Farias, *et al.*, (2022)	A he importance of nurses in providing self-care to patients with patients with Mellitus Type 1: a literature review. LILACS	Integrative review	The findings show that self-care and disease control reduce productivity losses and health costs, mainly by reducing complications, and are also associated with economic development.
03	Macedo *et al.*, (2024)	Self-care of adolescents with type 1 diabetes mellitus in Primary Health Care. LILACS	Descriptive, analytical a nd cross-sectional	It was observed in the study that difficulty in carrying out self-care practices predisposes to the emergence of complications such as retinopathy, neuropathy, nephropathy, cardiovascular disease and diabetic foot, reinforcing family support for adolescents in this process of change. Self-care is important to minimize and avoid these problems.

Continued from **Table 01** - Articles used in the systematic review.

NO.	Author/Year	Title/Databases	Type of study	Relevant results
04	Zanatta, Scaratti, Argenta, et al., (2020)	Experiences of adolescents with type 1 diabetes mellitus. BDENF	Qualitative study	The results of the study show that knowledge about the disease can lead to a positive self-perception that enables adolescents to build self-efficacy, which results in greater safety in managing diabetes and overcoming fear and situations of prejudice present in their environment.
05	Quinones; Geisler; Ramos, (2023)	The importance of Self-care in Patients with Diabetes Mellitus. LILACS	Literature lit erature	The findings show that in order to prevent diabetes-related morbidity and mortality, there is an immense need dedicated self-care behaviors in multiple domains, including dietary choices, physical activity, adequate medication intake and monitoring of patients' blood glucose.
06	Alves, Maia, Araújo, *et al.*, (2021)	Development and validation of a MHEALTH technology for promoting of self-care of adolescents with diabetes. BDENF	Experimental study	The study reports that the empowerment of adolescents with DM1 is, in fact, essential for keeping the disease under control and avoiding the main complications.
07	Marques, Coutinho, Martins, *et al.*, (2019)	Educational intervention for promotin g of self-care of elderly people with diabetes mellitus. BDENF	Experimental study	The study found that educational interventions for patients with diabetes favored positive attitudes towards the treatment and control of the disease, especially with regard to following a healthy diet.
08	Sá, Santana, Santos, *et al.*, (2023)	Educational technologies used for promotion of self-care of people with diabetes mellitus: integrative review. BDENF	Integrative literature review	This study reports that the focus of health education content is on promoting foot care, preventing neuropathy, self-management, knowledge and expectations of people with diabetes and preventing acute complications.

Continued from **Table 01** - Articles used in the systematic review.

NO.	**Author/Year**	**Title/Databases da tabases**	**Type of study**	**Relevant results**
09	Batista, Silva, Nóbrega *et al.*, (2021)	Adolescents with type 1 diabetes mellitus and the process of building autonomy for self-care. MEDLINE	Descriptive-exploratory research	As described in the study, the process of building the autonomy of adolescents with diabetes begins with their interest in seeking knowledge about the disease and treatment, enhanced by the support of their social network, boosting their self-confidence to take charge of their self-care.
10	Hermes, Rodrigues, Fonseca, *et al.*, (2021)	Repercussions of educational practice on self-care and management of type 1 Diabetes Mellitus in childhood. MEDLINE	Qualitative study	According to the study, physical activity proved to be an effective alternative for practicing self-care, but there was resistance to adopting eating habits aimed at diabetes, which are related to inadequate glycemic control and an increase in complications.
11	Oliveira, Batista, Camargos, *et al.*, (2022)	The influence of self-care and sources of social support on the management of type 1 diabetes mellitus. MEDLINE	Literature review	It can be understood that self-care is a fundamental component in the management of DM1, as it encourages the person's involvement in their treatment and greater adherence to the therapeutic regimen, minimizing complications and disabilities associated with chronic problems.
12	Silva, Costa, Santos, *et al.*, (2024)	The benefits of self-care protocols for patients with diabetes mellitus: a literatu re review. MEDLINE	Systematic review	In summary, the study is not only important for the prevention and control of DM, but is also fundamental for adherence to treatment, reduction of DM complications and significant health outcomes.

Source: Author.

The results of this study show that the importance of self-care for individuals with DM1 is based on preventing health problems, reducing health risks, reducing health service costs, improving patients' quality of life and minimizing health complications. This self-care involves physical activity, glycemic control, diet correction, self-efficacy, seeking professional support and understanding the information offered in health education.

Studies by Alves, *et al.* (2021), report that the empowerment of adolescents with DM1 is essential to keep the disease under control, avoiding the main complications. The study also mentions that insulin administration also presents challenges. For them, those with type I diabetes must carefully calculate insulin doses based on various factors, such as dietary intake and physical activity. Errors in these calculations can lead to dangerous episodes of hypoglycemia or hyperglycemia. In addition, the need for multiple daily injections or the constant use of an insulin pump can cause physical discomfort and emotional stress.

Furthermore, according to Quinones, Geisler & Ramos (2023), a balanced diet and carbohydrate control require constant planning and vigilance. Type I diabetes sufferers need to pay close attention to what they eat and how it affects their blood sugar levels. This can be especially difficult in social situations, such as eating out or attending events, where control over eating can be limited and social pressure can impede the need for discipline.

Another important obstacle for Macedo, *et al.* (2024) is regular physical exercise. For the author, although exercise has a positive effect on blood sugar control, it can also cause unexpected fluctuations in blood sugar levels. This requires careful planning and constant adjustments to insulin doses and diet before, during and after physical activity, which can be daunting and difficult to manage. In this sense, adherence to prescribed medication can be difficult due to the complexity of insulin and other medication regimes. Frequent adjustments and regular visits to the doctor are required, which can be logistically complicated and financially costly, especially for communities with limited access to health resources.

Macedo *et al.* (2024) also observed that the difficulty in carrying out self-care practices predisposes to the appearance of complications such as retinopathy, neuropathy, nephropathy, cardiovascular diseases and diabetic foot, reinforcing family support for adolescents in this process of change. Self-care is important to minimize and avoid these problems.

In this context, Alves, *et al.* (2021) corroborates the study by stating that foot care is an area that is often overlooked, but it is important to prevent serious complications. People with type I diabetes may have neuropathy and poor circulation, which increases the risk of foot injuries. Checking your feet every day and taking precautions can be a tedious task, and a little negligence can lead to serious problems such as ulcers and infections. Recognizing and responding to acute complications such as diabetic ketoacidosis requires a high level of knowledge and preparation. Lack of adequate information about the disease and its symptoms can cause serious delays in treatment, resulting in serious complications (Hermes, *et al.,* 2021). Studies carried out by Silva, *et al.* (2024). On the benefits of self-care protocols for patients with diabetes mellitus, a literature review states that a self-care program can be especially difficult for children and adolescents with type I diabetes, who may have difficulty accepting the disease and the need to differentiate themselves from their peers. Parents and caregivers also face challenges when trying to balance support and supervision with encouraging adolescent's independence. Furthermore, according to Oliveira, *et al.* (2022), self-care is the practice of actions carried out by individuals for their own benefit and to achieve quality of life. These are personal behaviors that can affect their health and well-being. However, this occurs simultaneously with environmental, social, economic, hereditary and health factors.

In this sense, the practice of self-care is an important part of the treatment of chronic diseases, such as DM1, as it allows the individual to observe and recognize symptoms, determine their aggressiveness and choose appropriate strategies to reduce these symptoms, thus maximizing their health. Promoting self-care has a positive impact on the treatment of DM1 because, by increasing the person's involvement in treatment, it can contribute to greater adherence and, consequently, reduce complications and disabilities associated with the problems caused by the disease (Oliveira, *et al.,* 2022).

Another study by Batista, *et al.* (2021), reports that the need for self-care to develop an effective DM1 treatment plan is related to knowledge of disease management, family support and its implications for the development of self-care, support from a multidisciplinary team and a support network.

In this sense, Marques, *et al.* (2019) educational actions represent a partnership between patients and educators (health professionals) aimed at self-care. These measures aim to involve patients in treatment decisions, making them managers of their disease and encouraging them to use the health system as a control tool when necessary. In this way, the educational process increases patient autonomy

In the studies by Almeida, Santos & Santos (2023) on the importance of diabetes education for patient self-care, they state that diabetes education is important as a strategy for increasing patient autonomy and self-care. The authors also report on the relationship between diabetes education and the adoption of healthy practices. In this sense, continuing education is essential to inform professionals about the new technologies and treatments available for DM. The rapid evolution of scientific evidence in this area makes it important for professionals to be informed in order to provide the best care for patients.

In addition, Quinones, Geisler & Ramos (2023) believe that for this process to be successful, patients must actively participate in the learning process, everyone's knowledge must be respected and time and space must be guaranteed for the exchange of information. Another important aspect is to set personalized goals and build ongoing relationships with patients so that they take more responsibility for managing their illness.

According to Oliveira, *et al.* (2022), regular blood sugar monitoring is very important. DM1 sufferers need to check their blood sugar several times a day in order to adjust insulin doses and avoid episodes of hypoglycemia (glucose levels that are too low) or hyperglycemia (glucose levels that are too high), both of which are potentially dangerous. In this sense, insulin administration is another important part of self-care. This is because people with type I diabetes need exogenous insulin to survive. This can be done through several daily injections or an insulin pump, which is a device that delivers insulin continuously.

Studies by Hermes, *et al.* (2021) report that a balanced and healthy diet also plays an important role. For them, carbohydrate control is necessary to avoid blood sugar spikes and maintain energy stability. Therefore, meal planning and carbohydrate counting are important practices for glycemic control. In addition to diet, regular exercise contributes significantly to controlling blood sugar levels. In this context, physical activity increases insulin sensitivity and helps reduce blood sugar levels. However, careful planning is needed to avoid hypoglycemia during or after exercise.

According to Araújo, *et al.* (2022) adequate hydration cannot be ignored. On the other hand, dehydration can have a negative impact on blood sugar levels. It is therefore important for people with type I diabetes to stay well hydrated, especially during physical activity or in hot weather. Another important aspect is foot care, as people with type I diabetes are more prone to foot problems due to poor circulation and neuropathy. In this context, checking the feet daily and wearing suitable footwear are important preventative measures to avoid injuries and infections (Sá*, et al., 2023).*

The study by Zanatta, *et al.* (2020) states that faced with an incurable disease, adolescents become more attentive and alert to possible complications, monitoring blood glucose levels, repeated insulin injections and other nutritional needs. In this sense, they gradually begin to accept new responsibilities previously attributed to the mother or the care team. According to Oliveira, *et al.* (2022), the support that adolescents receive in developing new self-care skills is fundamental to achieving autonomy and independence in the management of DM1.

In this sense, the study suggests the hypothesis that by acquiring new self-care skills, adolescents lose anxiety and gain confidence in self-administering insulin and regulating blood sugar levels.

CONCLUSION

From this study, it is understood that knowing the importance of self-care in coping with DM1 is fundamental due to the complexity and constant demands that this condition places on individuals. A complete understanding of self-care allows patients to be in a better condition and to make informed decisions regarding their daily care. This includes the correct administration of insulin, careful monitoring of glucose levels and the adoption of a healthy lifestyle, all of which are important factors for effective control of the disease.

The results of the studies analyzed allow us to answer the guiding question of this study - what is the impact of self-care on the health of individuals with DM1? In response to this question, it can be seen that self-care has a significant economic impact, as research shows that effective management of the disease can reduce the incidence of serious complications, which often require expensive treatments and can result in patients being hospitalized for long periods of time. Therefore, investing in education and support for self-care can result in significant savings for the healthcare system and improve patient outcomes.

In addition, understanding the importance of self-care helps to identify and overcome the barriers that individuals face in managing type 1 diabetes. These barriers can include lack of knowledge, access to quality medical services, emotional and psychological challenges.

We can highlight that research in this area can provide valuable information to better support patients by providing contextually appropriate resources and cultural interventions.

This study is therefore relevant and essential for the education and training of health professionals. Doctors, nurses and other professionals need to know the best self-care practices in order to effectively guide and support their patients. In addition to technical knowledge, communication skills are needed to motivate and encourage patients to adhere to their treatment plans.

In this context, learning the importance of self-care in DM1 encourages a holistic approach to the treatment of this disease. This includes not only managing the physical aspects of diabetes, but also the psychological and social support needed to help patients overcome the daily challenges of living with a chronic disease. In this way, an integrated and comprehensive self-care approach can result in improved quality of life and overall well-being for people with DM1.

In this sense, it is recommended that more studies be carried out on the subject in order to facilitate understanding of the topic and better disseminate knowledge about self-care in cases of DM1. In addition to the barriers and ways of encouraging self-care, the study can contribute to improving the approach of health professionals, the preparation of academics and the community's understanding of the subject.

REFERENCES

ALMEIDA, D.V.; SANTOS, J.C.; SANTOS, W.L. The importance of diabetes education for patient self-care. **Revista JRG de Estudos Acadêmicos**, v. 6, n. 13, p. 1664-1676, 2023.

ALVES, L.F.P.A.; MAIA, M.M.; ARAÚJO, M.F.M. *et al.* Development and validation of a MHEALTH technology to promote self-care in adolescents with diabetes. **Ciência & Saúde Coletiva**, v. 26, p. 1691-1700, 2021.

ARAÚJO, J. I. X; MELO, Y.S. FARIAS, J.R.T. *et al.* The importance of nurses in providing self-care to patients with type 1 diabetes mellitus: a literature review. **Revista Eletrônica Acervo Saúde**, V. 15, e. 9978, 2022.

BATISTA, A.F.M.; SILVA, M.E.; NÓBREGA, V.M. *et al.* Adolescents with type 1 diabetes mellitus and the process of building autonomy for self-care. **Revista de Enfermagem Referência**, n. 8, 2021.

BRITO, E.S.; PINTO, M.H., BERETTA, D. *et al.* Association between diabetes mellitus and eye diseases in visually impaired people. **Revista Enfermagem UERJ**,
v. 28,e49109, 2020.

CARDOSO NETO, C. A; OLIVEIRA, S. M. Impacto da educação biopsicossocial na qualidade de vida do idoso: revisão sistemática. **Research, Society and Development,** v. 12, n. 6,e13712642152, 2023.

DIXE, M.A.C.R.; GORDO, C.M.G.D.O.; CATARINO, H.B.P, *et al.* Effects of a education program in the knowledge and self-perception of school educators in preparing to care for type 1 diabetic children. **Einstein**, v. 18, p. 01-06, 2020.

DUTRA, A.R.B.; ALVES, L.O., AVENDANO, R.D.M.O. *et al.* Validation of educational-therapeutic technology applied to children with type 1 diabetes mellitus: standard institutional protocol. **Revista de Enfermagem da UFSM**, v. 13, e39, 2023.

GUZMAN O.A. **Case report: progression of chronic kidney disease in a**

diabetic patient. Course Conclusion Paper [Residency in Nephrology], 30 p. São Paulo: Hospital do Servidor Público Municipal, 2021.

HERMES, T.S.V; RODRIGUES, R. M ; FONSECA, L. M. M; TOSO, B. R. G. O; CONTERNO, S. F. R; VIERA, C. S. Repercussões da prática educativa no autocuidado e manejo do Diabetes Mellitus tipo 1 na infância. **Revista de Enfermagem da UFSM**, e.50, 2021.

JESUINO, A.G.A. A **importância do técnico de enfermagem na adaptação da família após diagnóstico da diabetes tipo I**. Course Conclusion Paper [Nursing Technician], 13 p. Porto Alegre: Escola Técnica GHC, 2021.

MACEDO, E.R.; SILVA N. C. R.; LAGO, K. D. S.; BARBONE, F. G. I.; CÉCILIO, A. O.
H. C.; SOUZA, D. A. Self-care of adolescents with type 1 diabetes mellitus in Primary Health Care. **Saúde (Santa Maria)**, v. 50, n. 1, 2024.

MARQUES, M.B.; COUTINHO, J.F.V.; MARTINS, M.C.; LOPES, M.V.D.O. *et al.* Educational intervention to promote self-care in the elderly with diabetes mellitus. **Revista da Escola de Enfermagem da USP**, v. 53, e03517, 2019.

MELO, E.G.; SANTOS, C.L.J. ; BATISTA-FILHO, R.A.; SOUZA, L.L. *et al.* Profile sociodemographic and clinical characteristics of elderly people with diabetes. **Revista de Enfermagem UFPE online**, v. 13, n. 3, p. 707-714, 2019.

MENDONÇA, J.A.; OLIVEIRA, D.; TEIXEIRA, A.S.; BRANDÃO, M.G.S.A. *et al.* Effectiveness of educational workshops on diabetic foot prevention for community health agents. **Revista Enfermagem Atual In Derme**, v. 96, n. 39, 2022.

MERINO, M.F.G.; SHIBUKAWA, B.M.C.; RISSI, G.P.; FONSECA, B.S.D. *et al.* Children and adolescents with diabetes: educational actions in the development of self-care skills. **Nursing**, ed. Bras. Impres., p. 8700-8713, 2022.

MOHER, D. *et al.* Preferred reporting items for systematic reviews and meta-analyses: the PRISMA statement. **PLoS Medicine**, v.6, n.7, e1000097, 2009.

NASS, E.M.A.; MARCON, S.S.; TESTON, E.F.; HADDAD, M.D.C.F.L. *et al.*

Psychosocial self-efficacy in young people with Diabetes Mellitus and its influence on self-care. **Revista Rene**, v. 20, e41412, 2019.

OLIVEIRA, R.E.S.; BATISTA, A.L.F.; CAMARGOS, B.S.R.; OLIVEIRA, E.L.F. *et al.* A
influence of self-care and sources of social support on the management of type 1 diabetes mellitus. **Revista Eletrônica Acervo Saúde**, v. 15, n. 11, e11043, 2022.

WHO. **Number of people with diabetes in the Americas more than triples in three decades, says PAHO report**. Geneva: World Health Organization, 2022. Available at: https://www.paho.org/pt/noticias/11-11-2022-numero-pessoas- com-diabetes-nas-americas-more-than-triples-in-three-decades#:~:text=A%20diabetes%20type%201%20occurs,by%20doen%C3%A7a % 20isqu%C3%AAmica%20do%20cora%C3%A7%C3%A3o. Accessed on July 2, 2024.

PEDRINHO, L.R.; SHIBUKAWA, B.M.C.; RISSI, G.P.; UEMA, R.T.B. *et al.* Brinquedo
therapy for children with type I diabetes mellitus: interventions at home.
Anna Nery School, v. 25, e20200278, 2020.

GUINONES, B.A.; GEISLER, S.A.; RAMOS, S. Importance of Self-Care in Patients with Diabetes Mellitus. **JRG Journal of Academic Studies**, v. 6, n. 13, p. 2057-2065, 2023.

RAMALHO, E L.R.; SPARAPANI, V.D.C.; BARBER, R.O.L.B.; OLIVEIRA, R.C. *et al.*
Clinical and sociodemographic factors associated with the quality of life of children and adolescents with type 1 diabetes. **Revista da Escola de Enfermagem da USP**, v. 57, e20230195, 2024.

REIS, H.M.; SILVA, G.L.; CAMPOS, W.B.S.; SILVEIRA, M.A.A. *et al.* Profile Epidemiology of Patients with Type 1 Diabetes Mellitus in the State of Sergipe between 2002 and 2012. **Revista Sergipana de Saúde Pública**, v. 2, n. 2, p. 25-35, 2023.

RODRIGUES, V.P.; MATOS, L.R.; TENANI, C.F. *BATISTA, M J.* Health literacy in diabetic adults using public health services in municipalities in São Paulo. **Revista de Ciências Médicas**, v. 31, p. 1-12, 2022.

ROSA, L.M.; IRMÃO, B.A.; BREHMER, L.C.; ANDRADE, A.E. *et al.* Bedside nursing
consultation and nursing diagnoses in people with diabetes mellitus. **Revista de Pesquisa Cuidado é Fundamental Online**, v. 13, p. 1436-1441, 2021.

SÁ, J.S.; SANTANA, M.D.O.; SANTOS, M.G.D.; BENEDITO, J.C.D.S. *et al.* Educational technologies used to promote self-care in people with diabetes mellitus: an integrative review. **Revista Brasileira de Enfermagem**, v. 76, p. e20230049, 2023.

SANTOS, A.L.; MARCON, S.S.; TESTON, E.F.; BACK, I.R. *et al.* Adherence to the treatment of diabetes mellitus and its relationship with primary care.
REME - Revista Mineira de Enfermagem, v. 24, e-1279, 2020.

SANTOS, M.M.C. **Training school health nurses to support children and young people with Type 1 Diabetes Mellitus**. Doctoral Thesis [Community Health Nursing], 215 p. Leiria/PT: Escola Superior de Saúde de Leiria, 2023.

SILVA, C.C.; COSTA, J.D.S.; SANTOS, J.K.; SILVA, N.C.N. *et al.* The benefits of the
self-care protocols for patients with diabetes mellitus: a literature review.
Multidisciplinary Journal Pey Këyo Científico, v. 10, n. 2, 2024.

SILVA, L.C.S.; SILVA, S.L.B.; OLIVEIRA, Á.M.S.D.; ARAÚJO, J.R.D. *et al.* Waistline
hypertriglyceridemia and associated factors in children and adolescents with type 1 diabetes mellitus. **Revista Paulista de Pediatria**, v. 38, e2019073, 2020.

SMANIOTTO, V.; PASCOLAT, G. The impact of type 1 diabetes mellitus on pediatric patients: analysis through drawings. **Revista Médica do Paraná**, v. 80, n. 1, p. 1702-1702, 2022.

SOUZA, R.R.; MARQUETE, V.F.; VIEIRA, V.C.; FISCHER, M.J.B. *et al.* Home care for child and adolescent home care with type 1 diabetes mellitus from the care giver's perspective. **Revista Enfermagem UERJ**, v. 28, e46013, 2020.

URRÚTIA, G.; BONFILL, X. PRISMA statement: a proposal to improve the publication of systematic reviews and metaanalyses. **Med Clin (Barc)**, v. 135, n. 11, p. 507-511, 2010.

ZANATTA, E.A.; SCARATTI, M.; ARGENTA, C.; BARICHELLO, A. Experiences of adolescents with type 1 diabetes mellitus. **Revista de Enfermagem Referência**, n. 4, 2020.

AUTHORS' BIOGRAPHIES

JANAICE VITÓRIA DIAS LIMA

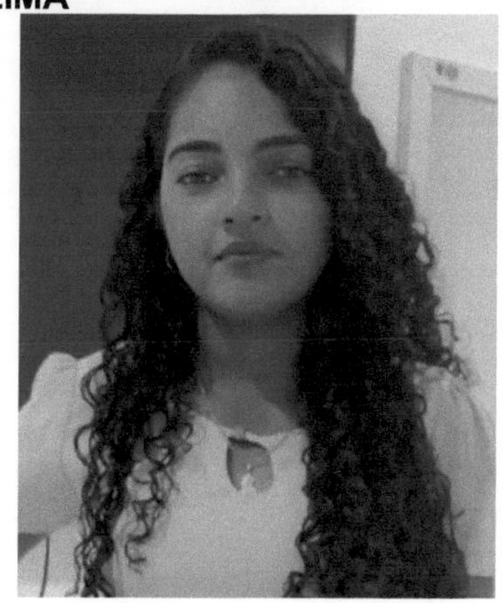

Bachelor's Degree in Nursing from Santa Luzia College-FSL. Nursing technician at the Santa Luzia Technical School of Commerce. Has expertise in Primary Care. Conducts health research.

ANTONIO DA COSTA CARDOSO NETO

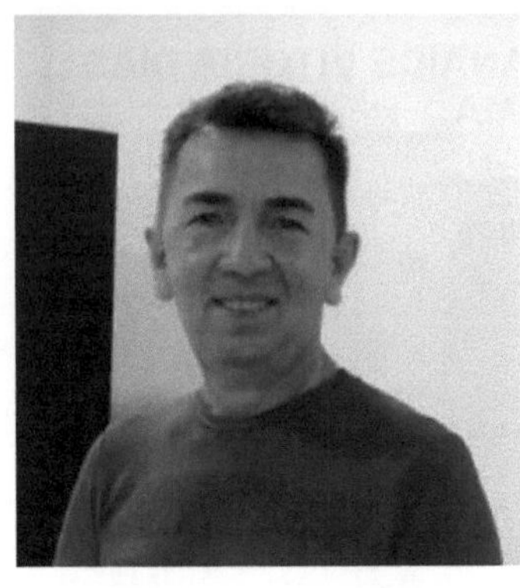

Post-Doctorate in Psychology from the University of Flores
- Buenos Aires / Argentina (2023). PhD in Collective Health from the Federal University of Maranhão - UFMA (2021). PhD in Public Health Sciences from the Universidad de Ciencias Empresariales y Sociales - UCES, Buenos Aires / Argentina (2018). Specialist in School Administration from Universidade Cândido Mendes/ RJ (2010). Specialist in Elderly Health from Estácio de Sá University/RJ (2011). Graduated in Nursing from Universidade CEUMA / MA (2008). Graduated in Pedagogy from the State University of Maranhão - UEMA (2001). He works as the Coordinator of Postgraduate Research and Extension, Professor of Scientific Methodology and Member of the Structuring Professor of the Nursing course at Faculdade Santa Luzia -FSL (2017 - current), teacher of Basic Education in the public education network of the Municipality of Santa Inês/Maranhão (1998 - current). He has been Coordinator of the Undergraduate Nursing Course since its creation (2012-2018), Academic Director (2018-2023), Institutional Prosecutor (PI) (2017-2023) and Institutional Researcher -CENSUP (2018) at Faculdade Santa Luzia -FSL. He was coordinator and teacher of technical courses at the Santa Luzia Technical School of Commerce - ETCSL / Maranhão (1996-2017). Assistant researcher at the Federal University of Maranhão
-UFMA (2006-2008). Researcher and Principal Sponsor of the Project: Biopsychosocial Education and Quality of Life for the Elderly. He has experience in drawing up Pedagogical Projects for Undergraduate Courses and drawing up Institutional Development Plans (PDI) Contacts: (098) 981090921. E-mail: cardosoneto.acc@gmail.com; cardosonetofsl2018@outlook.com.br. ORCID: https://orcid.org/0000-0003-3771-2821

MÁRCIA SILVA DE OLIVEIRA

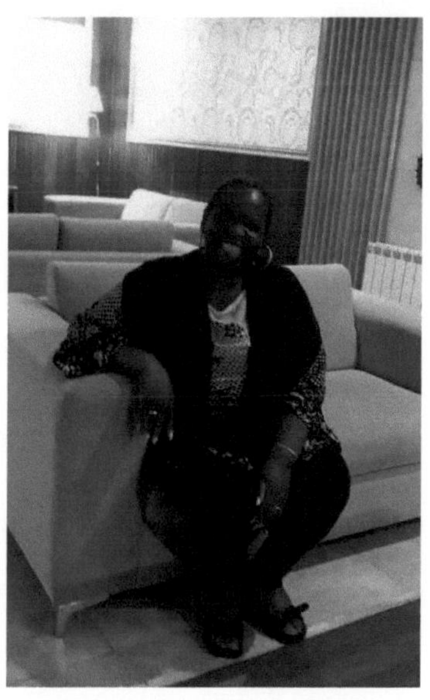

Post-Doctorate in Psychology - University of Flores (UFLO), Argentina. PhD in Public Health Sciences - Universidad de Ciencias Empresariales y Sociales (UCES), Argentina. Collaborating researcher at CITAB - Center for Research and Agro-environmental and Biological Technologies at the University of Trás-os-Montes and Alto Douro/Portugal. Master's Degree in Health Sciences - University of Brasília (UnB). Postgraduate in Clinical Analysis (Cytopathology) - São Judas Tadeu College/RJ. Postgraduate in Pathology - Castelo Branco University/RJ. Postgraduate in University Teaching (Research Methodology and Pedagogical Research and Practice) - UniCEUB/DF. Graduated in Biological Sciences - Medical Modality (Biomedicine) from the State University of Rio de Janeiro (Anatomy). General/Pedagogical Coordinator of the Brasília Campus of Universidade Paulista (UNIP/Brasília). Professor of Pathology, Immunology, Didactics Applied to Nursing, Educational Practice in Health and Integrating Seminar of the Nursing course at Faculdade Santa Luzia (FSL)/Santa Inês/MA. Lecturer with experience in organizing, participating in, coordinating, planning and monitoring health and education projects, both inside and outside pedagogical learning spaces. Good interpersonal relationships, responsibility and dedication to work activities. Biomedical Supervisor at Laboratório Médico Dr. Maricondi Ltda (WAMA Diagnóstica), São Carlos/SP (Costa Verde Unit - Itaguaí/RJ). Lecturer in Safety, Environment and Health and Quality Management System at the Rio de Janeiro State Technical School Support Foundation (FAETEC/RJ) Lecturer on undergraduate courses in Medicine, Dentistry, Nursing, Veterinary Medicine and Architecture and Urbanism at the Faculdades Integradas do Planalto Central (FACIPLAC/DF). Lecturer on undergraduate courses in Biomedicine, Physiotherapy, Psychology, Biological Sciences and Mathematics at Universidade Paulista (UNIP - Campus Brasília). Coordinator and lecturer on postgraduate and extension courses at the Instituto Educacional Evangélico do Centro-Oeste - UNIECO/DF. Lecturer in Hormonology on the Postgraduate course in Clinical, Toxicological and Bromatological Analysis at the Instituto Brasil Pesquisa e Extensão - IBEP. Full Researcher at the Center for Studies in Health Promotion and Inclusive Projects at the University of Brasília - NESPROM/UnB.

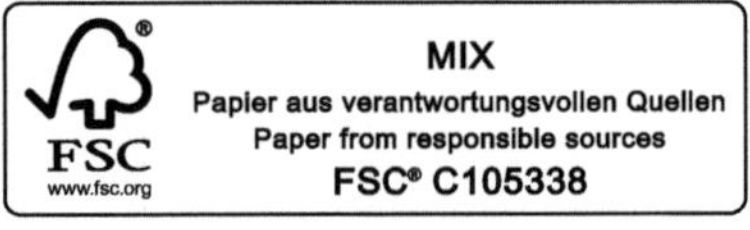

Printed by Books on Demand GmbH, Norderstedt / Germany